W9-BJN-775

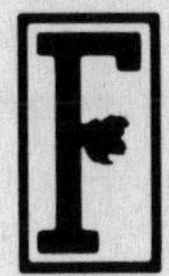

EARL MINDELL IS ALSO THE AUTHOR OF:

Earl Mindell's Herb Bible

Earl Mindell's Food as Medicine

Earl Mindell's
Soy Miracle Cookbook

70 Simple, Tasty Ways to Add Soy Protein to Your Diet

Earl Mindell, R.Ph., Ph.D.

RECIPES FROM

Earl Mindell's
Soy Miracle

A FIRESIDE BOOK
Published by Simon & Schuster
New York London Toronto Sydney Tokyo Singapore

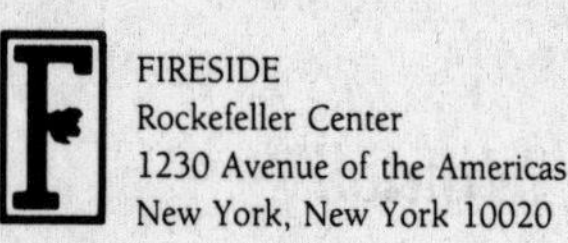

FIRESIDE
Rockefeller Center
1230 Avenue of the Americas
New York, New York 10020

Manufactured in the United States of America

10 9 8 7 6 5 4 3 2

Library of Congress Cataloging-in-Publication Data is available

ISBN: 0-684-82607-0

The recipes in this book were previously published in *Earl Mindell's Soy Miracle*, copyright © 1995 by Earl Mindell, R.Ph., Ph.D. and Carol Colman.

Acknowledgments

I wish to express my deep and lasting appreciation to the people who have assisted me in this book, especially Bonny Redlich, a superb researcher; Judith Eaton, M.S., R.D., and Karen Lefkowitz, M.S., for their wonderful recipes; Sherry Wehner of Protein Technologies, Int., St. Louis; the Soyfoods Association of America and the United Soybean Board for their help; and all the soyfood producers mentioned in this book. In addition, I would like to thank all of the soybean researchers in the United States and throughout the world from whose work we all benefit. Finally, special thanks to Josh Gerber for his fine proofreading, to my editors Marilyn Abraham and Sheila M. Curry for their wise advice and assistance, and to Philip Metcalf and Carole Berglie for their help with copyediting and production. Much thanks to Richard Curtis, my agent, for his help throughout the years.

Introduction

Want to know how to get more soy into your life? This book contains seventy recipes for appetizers, soups, main courses, and desserts—all based on soy products and all good tasting. Many of these recipes were developed by nutritionists Judith Eaton, M.S., R.D., and Karen Lefkowitz, M.S., who, as they say, have been carrying the tofu torch for many years. Judith and Karen run Nutrition Services, a consulting firm in Pomona, New York, with clients ranging from industry to private patients. Judith is the prenatal nutrition consultant for Phelps Memorial Hospital in New York and for Planned Parenthood, and a nutrition consultant for the American Health Foundation. Karen is a nutrition consultant for the

Child Health Center of the American Health Foundation. She has also served as a consultant for the Pediatric Department of New York Medical College. Judith and Karen have devoted a great deal of their professional time to solving the nutritional problems of children and teenagers. They are coordinators of the American Health Foundation's Bodybeat Program, a weight-management program for young adolescents and have worked with children with high cholesterol.

In order to reduce fat, Judith and Karen use Mori-Nu brand's low-fat tofu in their recipes. If you substitute other tofus, remember it will add a few more fat grams and calories. (A 4-ounce serving of regular firm tofu contains 6 grams of fat and 120 calories; regular soft tofu contains 5 fat grams and 86 calories; regular silken tofu contains 2.4 fat grams and 72 calories.)

I have also collected terrific recipes from other sources. Macrobiotic cook Ana McIntyre, a well-known spa chef, contributed three of her unique soy recipes.

Lynne Paterson, product development consultant to Lightlife Foods, is an internationally recognized cooking teacher, caterer, and frequent contributor to *Natural Health Magazine*. Ms. Paterson, a professional chef and owner of Valley Natural Foodservices of Shutesbury, Massachusetts, contributed an original soyfood recipe to this book. In addition, some soy food producers were kind enough to share their best recipes.

Several producers of high-quality soyfood products, including Vitasoy, Eden Foods, Azumaya, Bountiful Bean Soyfoods, and Worthington Foods (marketed under the brand name Natural Touch) also contributed some excellent recipes. Their products can be found at natural food stores and many supermarkets. In addition, we received some terrific recipes from the Soyfoods Association of America, the United Soybean Board, the Missouri Soybean Board, and Soy Ohio. Many of these soyfood manufacturers and trade associations will provide additional recipes free of charge.

In some recipes, we specify that a low-fat or no-fat version of a particular ingredient, or a no-salt or salt-reduced ingredient, is preferred. Keep in mind that the nutritional analysis is based on the lowest fat, lowest salt product. In addition, we did not include optional ingredients, or optional accompaniment such as bread, crackers, or chips, in the analysis. Unless otherwise specified, use medium-size fruits and vegetables in the recipes.

The Recipes

Salads *15*

Curried Tofu Rice Salad 15
Vegetable Couscous with Tofu 17
Tofu Mock Egg Salad 18
Tempeh Mock Chicken Salad 19

Spreads, Dressings, and Sauces *20*

Peanut Butter and Jelly Lover's Tofu Spread 20
Tofu Tuna Spread 21
Savory Cheese Spread 22
Herbed Tofu Pâté 23
Tofu Ginger-Peanut Dressing 24
Sweet Poppy Dressing 25
Tofu Mole Dip 26
Zesty Cilantro Dip 27
Creamy White Sauce 28
Cholesterol-Free Hollandaise Sauce 29

Soups *30*

Cream of Cauliflower Soup 30
Spicy Carrot Soup 31
Crabmeat and Asparagus Soup 33
Tofu and Corn Bisque 34
Cream of Vegetable Soup 35
Miso Soup with Onions 36

Main Dishes *37*

Tofu Sloppy Joes 37
Sloppy Joes with Texturized Soy Protein 39
Fusilli and Tofu with Sauce Verde 40
Tofu Meatballs 41
Tofu Cutlets Parmesan 42
Tofu Stuffed Pepper 43
Quinoa with Tofu 45
Crustless Onion-Mushroom Quiche 46
Athenian Tofu 47
Okara Patties with Spicy Peanut Sauce 48
Okara Patty Foo Yong 49
Tempeh Pizza 50
Busy Day Chili 51
Sweet-and-Sour Hawaiian Tempeh 52
Quick-and-Easy Spinach Lasagna 53
Tempeh Reuben Sandwiches 55
Barbecued Tofu 56
Tofu with Condiments 57
Sesame Tofu 58
Noodle Pudding 59

Tempeh-Lemon Broil 60
Barbecued Grilled Tempeh with Onions 61
Tex-Mex Tempeh 61
Rice and Tofu Loaf 63
Tofu and Mushrooms 64
Tofu Rice Stir-Fry 65
Tofu Bouillabaisse 66
Chicken Tetrazzini 67
Chicken and Tofu Stir-Fry 69
Chicken Paprika 70
Beefy Tofu Enchiladas 71
Meat Loaf 72

Breads and Breakfasts 73

Peach Breakfast Soufflé 73
Toffins 74
Zucchini Bread 75
Eastern Omelet 77
Apple Pancakes 78
Banana Pancakes 79

Desserts 80

Chocolate Tofu Berry Whip 80
Chocolate Chip Cookies 81
Chocolate Cream Pie 82
Tofu Brownies 83
Tofu Strawberry Cheese Cake 84
Creamy Spritzer 85

Tofu Pumpkin Pie 86
Strawberry Fluff 87
Super-Moist Carrot Cake 88
Vanilla Pudding 89
Piña Colada 90
Low Cal Chocolate Mousse 90

Salads

Curried Tofu Rice Salad

Serves 4

1 package (10½ ounces) firm or extra-firm low-fat tofu, drained

1½ cups cooked brown rice

2 scallions, finely chopped

1 tablespoon finely chopped fresh parsley

1 tomato, diced

DRESSING

½ tablespoon lemon juice

½ teaspoon curry powder

⅛ teaspoon chili powder

½ teaspoon garlic powder

¼ teaspoon salt

⅛ teaspoon ground black pepper

1 tablespoon olive oil

2½ tablespoons vinegar

GARNISH

Lettuce leaves
Sliced cucumbers
Sliced red and green bell peppers

1. Slice the tofu and drain between several layers of paper towels for 15 to 20 minutes. Remove tofu and crumble into small pieces and place in bowl. Add the rice, scallions, parsley, and tomato and mix well.

2. Mix seasonings for dressing with oil. Toss with tofu-rice mixture, then toss with vinegar. Let marinate from 30 minutes to several hours in the refrigerator.

3. Serve on lettuce leaves and garnish with slices of cucumbers and red and green peppers.

PER SERVING Calories: 154 | Fat: 5 g
Saturated fat: under 1 g | Fiber: 2 g
Cholesterol: 0 | Sodium: 209 mg
Calcium: 29 mg | Iron: 6 mg

RESOURCE: Judith Eaton and Karen Lefkowitz

Vegetable Couscous with Tofu

Serves 6

2 packages (10½ ounces each) extra-firm low-fat tofu
1 large onion, chopped
1 large red bell pepper, chopped
4 carrots, thinly sliced
2 zucchini, sliced in ½-inch pieces
1 can (15 ounces) navy beans, rinsed and drained
1½ cups tomato sauce, preferably low salt
1½ cups low-salt, fat-free chicken broth
½ cup raisins
2 teaspoons curry powder
¼ teaspoon cayenne pepper
1 teaspoon paprika
1¾ cups couscous

1. Cut the tofu into ½-inch cubes. Drain in colander.

2. Spray a heavy, large skillet with nonstick cooking spray. Add the onion, pepper, carrots, and tofu. Sauté for 10 minutes, stirring occasionally.

3. Add the zucchini and cook an additional 2 minutes.

4. Add the beans, tomato sauce, broth, raisins, curry powder, cayenne, and paprika. Cover and bring to boil. Simmer for 30 minutes.

5. Prepare couscous according to package directions. Serve cooked vegetables over couscous.

PER SERVING		
	Calories: 433	Fat: 2.5 g
	Saturated fat: under 2 g	Fiber: 12 g
	Cholesterol: 0	Sodium: 538 mg
	Calcium: 108 mg	Iron: 10.6 mg

RESOURCE: Judith Eaton and Karen Lefkowitz

Tofu Mock Egg Salad

Serves 4

1 pound firm tofu
1 tablespoon low-sodium soy sauce
¾ teaspoon prepared mustard
¼ teaspoon garlic powder
¼ teaspoon curry powder
Pinch of cayenne pepper
1 tablespoon minced fresh parsley
1 small celery stalk, chopped
1 tablespoon minced onion
2 tablespoons mayonnaise, preferably reduced-fat
2 tablespoons honey
1 tablespoon lemon juice

1. Mash the tofu with a fork in a large bowl.

2. Combine with remaining ingredients and mix well. Adjust seasonings to taste.

3. Spread on bread, toast or crackers, or serve as a vegetable dip.

PER SERVING (NOT INCLUDING ACCOMPANIMENTS)	Calories: 176	Fat: 7 g
	Saturated fat: 1 g	Fiber: less than 1 g
	Cholesterol: 2.5 mg	Sodium: 171 mg
	Calcium: 128 mg	Iron: 6.4 mg

RESOURCE: Bountiful Bean Soyfoods

Tempeh Mock Chicken Salad

Serves 2

1 cup water
8 ounces tempeh, cut in 1-inch pieces
1 bay leaf
1 tablespoon sesame tahini
1 tablespoon white miso
1 teaspoon prepared mustard
1 celery stalk, finely diced
¼ cup minced scallions

1. In a small saucepan, bring water to a boil. Add the tempeh and bay leaf. Cover, reduce heat, and simmer for about 20 minutes.

2. Remove the lid and boil off remaining water. Let tempeh cool.

3. In a bowl, mash the tempeh with the tahini, miso, and mustard. Mix in the celery and scallions. Refrigerate for several hours.

4. Serve as a side-dish salad on lettuce leaves or as a filling for sandwiches or pita pockets.

PER SERVING Calories: 270 Fat: 15 g
Saturated fat: less than 1 g Fiber: 5 g
Cholesterol: 0 Sodium: 377 mg
Calcium: 122 mg Iron: 3 mg

RESOURCE: Ana McIntyre

Spreads, Dressings, and Sauces

Peanut Butter and Jelly Lover's Tofu Spread

Serves 3

Love PB and J but hate the fat? Try this lower-fat version on bread or crackers.

1 package (10½ ounces) firm low-fat tofu
3 tablespoons natural-style chunky peanut butter
¼ cup black raspberry all-fruit preserves

1. Drain the tofu.

2. Place the tofu and peanut butter in a food processor and process until smooth.

3. Add the preserves and process with on/off motion until blended. Chill for several hours to allow flavors to blend.

PER SERVING	Calories: 180	Fat: 8 g
	Saturated fat: 1 g	Fiber: 1 g
	Cholesterol: 0	Sodium: 95 mg
	Calcium: 23 mg	Iron: 7 mg

RESOURCE: Judith Eaton and Karen Lefkowitz

Tofu Tuna Spread

Serve as a sandwich spread or with crackers and crudités.

Serves 4

1 package (10½ ounces) firm or extra-firm low-fat tofu
1 can (6⅛ ounces) tuna, packed in water
1 small purple onion
½ cup grated carrot
¼ cup chopped fresh parsley
1 tablespoon fat-free mayonnaise or soy mayonnaise
2 tablespoons honey mustard

1. Drain the tofu and tuna.

2. In a food processor, chop the onion.

3. Add the tofu and tuna and process until desired consistency. Stir in the carrots and parsley.

4. In a small bowl, mix the mayonnaise and mustard, then blend into the tuna mixture.

PER SERVING Calories: 84 | Fat: 2.5 g
Saturated fat: less than 1 g | Fiber: 1 g
Cholesterol: 5 g | Sodium: 106 mg
Calcium: 28 mg | Iron: 1 mg

RESOURCE: Judith Eaton and Karen Lefkowitz

Savory Cheese Spread

Makes 36 1-tablespoon servings

½ cup grated reduced-fat, low-salt cheddar cheese
½ cup grated Parmesan cheese
½ cup mashed tofu
½ cup mayonnaise, preferably reduced-fat
¼ cup diced pitted green olives
2 tablespoons grated onion
2 tablespoons chopped fresh parsley
1 teaspoon curry powder
Party rye slices

1. Combine all the ingredients in mixing bowl.
2. Spread on party rye and serve.

PER SERVING Calories: 24 | Fat: 2 g
Saturated fat: under 1 g | Fiber: 0
Cholesterol: 3 mg | Sodium: 58 mg
Calcium: 35 mg | Iron: less than 1 mg

RESOURCE: Missouri Soybean Board

Herbed Tofu Pâté

Makes 36 1-tablespoon servings

1 pound firm tofu, drained
1 tablespoon white miso
1 tablespoon sesame tahini
1 teaspoon umeboshi plum paste
1 teaspoon fresh lemon juice
1 tablespoon minced chives
1 tablespoon minced fresh basil

1. Drain excess water from the tofu by either slicing and pressing under a weight or wringing out in a clean cotton towel.

2. Place all ingredients in a mixing bowl and mash thoroughly until smooth.

3. Press the mixture into a mold and refrigerate for several hours or overnight to let the flavors blend.

4. Slice or scoop out and serve on sandwiches or crackers for a tasty, lower-fat alternative to a cream cheese spread.

PER SERVING	Calories: 14	Fat: 1 g
	Saturated fat: less than 1 g	Fiber: less than 1 g
	Cholesterol: 0	Sodium: 18 mg
	Calcium: 14 mg	Iron: less than 1 mg

RESOURCE: Ana McIntyre

Tofu Ginger-Peanut Dressing

This sauce is terrific on oriental chicken salad, raw veggies, steamed vegetables, or salad greens. Mix with whole wheat or buckwheat noodles for a lunch kids really enjoy. It will stay fresh in the refrigerator for up to one week.

Serves 12

3 scallions (white part only)
3-inch piece fresh ginger, peeled
2 garlic cloves
3 tablespoons natural-style peanut butter, smooth or chunky
2 packages (10½ ounces) firm low-fat tofu
1 teaspoon dark roasted sesame oil
⅓ cup low-sodium soy sauce
¼ cup honey
1 cup rice wine vinegar
2 cups water

1. Process the scallions, ginger, and garlic in a food processor or blender until smooth.

2. Add the peanut butter, tofu, sesame oil, soy sauce, and honey; process until the mixture is blended.

3. Slowly add the vinegar and water, and process until blended.

PER SERVING	Calories: 75	Fat: 2.5 g
	Saturated fat: under 1 g	Fiber: under 1 g
	Cholesterol: 12 mg	Sodium: 299 mg
	Calcium: 16 mg	Iron: 4 mg

RESOURCE: Judith Eaton and Karen Lefkowitz

Sweet Poppy Dressing

Serves 8

2 tablespoons Dijon-style mustard
2 tablespoons honey
Juice of 1 lemon
1 cup Light Original Vitasoy
2 teaspoons poppy seeds
½ teaspoon paprika
¼ teaspoon grated orange zest

1. Mix the mustard and honey in a bowl.

2. Slowly blend in the lemon juice and soy milk. Add the remaining ingredients.

3. Use to dress a crisp green salad or as a vegetable dip.

PER SERVING	Calories: 72	Fat: 3g
	Saturated fat: less than 1g	Fiber: 0
	Cholesterol: 0	Sodium: 629 mg
	Calcium: 46 mg	Iron: 0

RESOURCE: Vitasoy, Inc.

Tofu Mole Dip

Makes 37 1-tablespoon servings

1 package (10½ ounces) soft tofu, drained
1½ teaspoons lemon juice
1 teaspoon garlic powder
2 tablespoons diced onion
2 tablespoons chopped fresh cilantro
½ teaspoon chili powder
1 small tomato, diced
1 ripe medium avocado, mashed

1. In a blender or food processor, combine the tofu, lemon juice, garlic powder, onion, cilantro, and chili powder until well blended.

2. Put the mixture in a serving bowl. Add the tomato and avocado, and mix well. Chill and serve with no-fat chips or fresh vegetables.

PER SERVING	Calories: 19	Fat: 1 g
	Saturated fat: less than 1 g	Fiber: less than 1 g
	Cholesterol: 0	Sodium: 3 mg
	Calcium: 4.7 mg	Iron: less than 1 mg

RESOURCE: Missouri Soybean Board

Zesty Cilantro Dip

Serves 8

½ cup chopped fresh cilantro
1 can (4 ounces) green chilies, diced and drained
2 cups frozen petite peas, thawed
1 package (10½ ounces) low-fat firm tofu, drained
1 tablespoon lemon juice
1½ teaspoons ground cumin
¼ teaspoon freshly ground pepper
Salt to taste (optional)

2 tomatoes, sliced
4 cups sliced raw vegetables of choice

1. In a food processor or blender, combine ¼ cup cilantro and all the dip ingredients until smooth, blending approximately 30 seconds on high. Refrigerate for 1 hour.

2. Mound on overlapping tomato slices and rim with fresh cilantro. Serve with vegetables.

PER SERVING	Calories: 62 g	Fat: 1 g
	Saturated fat: less than 1 g	Fiber: 0
	Cholesterol: 0	Sodium: 50 mg
	Calcium: 30 mg	Iron: 1 mg

RESOURCE: Mori-nu

Creamy White Sauce

Serves 4

1 tablespoon vegetable oil
1½ tablespoons organic unbleached white flour
1½ cups Edensoy Original Organic soy milk
½ teaspoon sea salt
2 large garlic cloves, crushed
2 teaspoons mirin (rice wine)
2 tablespoons finely chopped fresh parsley

1. Mix the oil and flour in a heavy saucepan. Warm over low heat, stirring constantly, for 3 to 5 minutes. Slowly add the soy milk, stirring constantly as sauce thickens.

2. Add salt, garlic, and mirin. Simmer uncovered over low heat, stirring occasionally for 10 to 15 minutes. Remove from heat and stir in parsley.

3. Serve over pasta.

PER SERVING	Calories: 75	Fat: 9 g
	Saturated fat: less than 1 g	Fiber: less than 1 g
	Cholesterol: 0	Sodium: 280 mg
	Calcium: 11 mg	Iron: less than 1 mg

RESOURCE: Eden Foods

Cholesterol-Free Hollandaise Sauce

This eggless hollandaise is delicious over cooked vegetables, fish, tempeh, tofu, or seafood.

Serves 4

1 cup Edensoy Original Organic soy milk

2 tablespoons corn oil

¼ teaspoon sea salt

1 tablespoon kudzu or cornstarch, dissolved in 2 tablespoons water

1 tablespoon lemon juice

Paprika or ground nutmeg, for garnish

1. Combine the soy milk, oil, salt, and kudzu or cornstarch mixture in a saucepan. Simmer for 3 to 5 minutes, stirring constantly with wire whisk, until mixture becomes thick.

2. Add lemon juice to sauce, then pour over hot food. Garnish with paprika or nutmeg.

PER SERVING	Calories: 90	Fat: 8 g
	Saturated fat: less than 1 g	Fiber: 0
	Cholesterol: 0	Sodium: 140 mg
	Calcium: 4 mg	Iron: less than 1 mg

RESOURCE: Eden Foods

Soups

Cream of Cauliflower Soup

Serves 8

1 large cauliflower
2 teaspoons canola oil
1 onion, chopped
3 celery stalks, chopped
¼ cup all-purpose flour
4 cups fat-free, low-salt chicken broth, canned or homemade
1 package (10½ ounces) soft low-fat tofu
1 cup skim milk
1 teaspoon paprika
1 teaspoon grated nutmeg
Salt and pepper to taste (optional)
Grated Parmesan cheese, preferably fat-free cheese alternative (optional)

1. Cut the cauliflower into florets and remove stems. Steam lightly for 12 minutes or microwave on high for 5 to 7 minutes.

2. Drain the cauliflower and reserve about one third of the florets. Puree the remaining florets in a blender or food processor.

3. In a large pot, heat the oil and sauté the onion and celery until tender, about 5 minutes.

4. Add the flour to the vegetables and stir. Slowly add the chicken broth and bring to a boil. Mix in the pureed cauliflower and reduce heat to a simmer.

5. In a blender or food processor, blend the tofu and milk. Slowly add this mixture to soup.

6. Add the reserved florets, paprika, nutmeg, and optional salt and pepper. Pour into serving bowls and, if desired, add a sprinkling of Parmesan cheese.

PER SERVING		
	Calories: 97	Fat: 3 g
	Saturated fat: under 1 g	Fiber: 3 g
	Cholesterol: under 1 mg	Sodium: 235 mg
	Calcium: 83 mg	Iron: 1 mg

RESOURCE: Judith Eaton and Karen Lefkowitz

Spicy Carrot Soup

Serves 4

1 tablespoon olive oil
1 small onion, chopped
4 large carrots, chopped
1 garlic clove, minced
¼ teaspoon mustard seeds
¼ teaspoon ground ginger
¼ teaspoon ground cumin
¼ teaspoon turmeric
Pinch of ground cinnamon
Pinch of cayenne pepper
¼ teaspoon salt
½ tablespoon lemon juice

½ cup water

2 tablespoons unsalted margarine

2 tablespoons whole wheat flour

2 packages (16.8 ounces each) Creamy Original Vitasoy soy milk

½ teaspoon honey

¼ cup low-fat yogurt

1. In a large saucepan, heat the olive oil and sauté the onion until golden, about 3 minutes. Add the carrots, garlic, mustard seeds, spices, salt, and lemon juice. Cook for 2 to 3 minutes, stirring constantly.

2. Add the water, cover, and simmer for 20 minutes or until carrots are tender. Let cool.

3. Place the mixture in a blender and puree on low speed until smooth.

4. In a sauce pan, melt the margarine, add the flour, and cook for 2 to 3 minutes, stirring constantly. Whisk in the soy milk, then add the carrot puree and cook for 10 minutes, stirring constantly. Serve hot with a spoonful of yogurt on top.

PER SERVING	Calories: 182	Fat: 10 g
	Saturated fat: 2 g	Fiber: 3 g
	Cholesterol: 0	Sodium: 159 mg
	Calcium: 75 mg	Iron: less than 1 mg

RESOURCE: Vitasoy, Inc.

Crabmeat and Asparagus Soup

Serves 3

½ pound fresh asparagus

1 tablespoon unsalted margarine

¼ cup finely chopped onion

2 tablespoons whole wheat flour

2 packages (16.8 ounces) Creamy Original Vitasoy soy milk

¼ teaspoon salt

pinch each of black pepper, paprika, garlic powder, and ground nutmeg

½ pound fresh asparagus

¼ pound lump crabmeat

1. Wash the asparagus well. Steam until tender, about 15 minutes, then chop and drain.

2. In a large saucepan, melt the margarine over medium heat. Stir in onion and sauté until golden, about 3 minutes. Add the flour and cook the mixture for 2 to 3 minutes, stirring constantly.

3. Gradually whisk in the soy milk, then add the salt and other seasonings, stirring constantly.

4. Add the asparagus, reduce heat to low, and cook for 5 minutes.

5. Add the crabmeat and bring the soup to boil. Serve immediately.

PER SERVING		
	Calories: 175	Fat: 7 g
	Saturated fat: 1 g	Fiber: 2 g
	Cholesterol: 39 mg	Sodium: 370 mg
	Calcium: 84 mg	Iron: 1 mg

RESOURCE: Vitasoy, Inc.

Tofu and Corn Bisque

Serves 8

4 tablespoons unsalted margarine
2 small onions, finely chopped
2 teaspoons mild curry powder
2 teaspoons paprika
½ cup all-purpose flour
4 cups vegetable stock
1 package (33.8 ounces) Light Original Vitasoy soy milk
Grated rind of 1 lemon
1 large can (24 ounces) whole kernel corn, drained
1 package (16 ounces) firm tofu, drained and cubed
2 tablespoons chopped fresh parsley

1. Melt margarine in a large saucepan and gently cook the onions until soft, about 5 minutes.

2. Stir in the curry powder, paprika, and flour and cook for 1 minute. Gradually add the stock and bring to boil, stirring constantly.

3. Stir in the soy milk, lemon rind, and corn. Simmer for 5 minutes.

4. Stir in tofu and simmer for 5 minutes. Garnish with parsley.

PER SERVING	Calories: 386	Fat: 17 g
	Saturated fat: 3 g	Fiber: 3 g
	Cholesterol: 4 mg	Sodium: 626 mg
	Calcium: 191 mg	Iron: 8 mg

RESOURCE: Vitasoy, Inc.

Cream of Vegetable Soup

Any leftover vegetables can be used in this soup!

Serves 10

2 teaspoons olive oil
1 cup chopped onion
2 garlic cloves, minced
4 carrots, chopped
2 celery stalks, chopped
2 cups shredded green cabbage
1 can (2 pounds, 3 ounces) Italian-style plum tomatoes
4 cups fat-free, low-salt canned chicken broth, or 4 cups homemade chicken stock
2 tablespoons chopped fresh parsley, or 2 teaspoons dried
2 tablespoons chopped fresh dill, or 2 teaspoons dried
2 tablespoons chopped fresh basil, or 2 teaspoons dried
1 teaspoon dried oregano
1 tablespoon sugar
Salt and pepper to taste (optional)
1 package (10½ ounces) soft low-fat tofu

1. In a large, heavy pot, heat the olive oil over medium heat. Add the onions and garlic and cook for 3 minutes.

2. Add the carrots, celery, and cabbage and sauté briefly, 2 to 3 minutes.

3. Add the tomatoes and chicken broth. Stir in the parsley, dill, basil, oregano, sugar, and optional salt and pepper. Bring to boil, lower heat and simmer for 1 hour.

4. Carefully, 1 cup at a time, puree the soup in a blender or food processor. Return soup to pot.

5. Blend the tofu in a blender or food processor. Slowly add tofu to soup and mix well. Heat soup thoroughly.

PER SERVING	Calories: 84	Fat: 2.6 g
	Saturated fat: under 1 g	Fiber: 2.5 g
	Cholesterol: 0	Sodium: 322 mg
	Calcium: 64 mg	Iron: 1.5 mg

RESOURCE: Judith Eaton and Karen Lefkowitz

Miso Soup with Onions

Serves 4

4 cups water
1 cup sliced onion
1 low-sodium bouillon cube (chicken, vegetable, or beef)
1 package (10½ ounces) extra-firm low-fat tofu, diced
½ tablespoon low-sodium soy sauce
1 tablespoon dark miso, diluted in a little soup stock
½ cup nori *(dried seaweed)*
2 scallions, thinly sliced

1. Place the water in a large pot and bring to boil over medium heat. Add the onion and bouillon cube; simmer for 2 minutes.

2. Add the tofu and soy sauce; simmer 5 minutes.

3. Add the diluted miso and stir gently. Turn heat to low and simmer for 2 to 3 minutes.

4. Lightly toast the *nori* over an open flame or stove burner until the color changes; crumble and add to soup.

5. Serve and garnish with scallions.

PER SERVING	Calories: 65	Fat: 1 g
	Saturated fat: under 1 g	Fiber: 1.3 g
	Cholesterol: 0	Sodium: 399 mg
	Calcium: 43 mg	Iron: 6 mg

RESOURCE: Judith Eaton and Karen Lefkowitz

Main Dishes

Tofu Sloppy Joes

Serves 3

3 English muffins, preferably whole grain, split in halves
1 package (10½ ounces) soft or firm low-fat tofu, drained
½ cup fat-free, salt-reduced, meatless spaghetti sauce
1½ teaspoons grated Parmesan cheese
6 tablespoons shredded reduced-fat mozzarella, or reduced-fat soy cheese

1. Toast the muffins until lightly browned.

2. Place the tofu in a nonstick frying pan and mash with a potato masher or fork. Cook over high heat for 5 minutes, stirring occasionally.

3. Add the pasta sauce and continue cooking over high heat for 4 minutes, stirring occasionally.

4. Divide the tofu mixture among the 6 muffin halves and sprinkle each with ¼ teaspoon Parmesan cheese.

5. Top each with a tablespoon of mozzarella cheese.

6. Place on a microwave-safe plate and cook on high in microwave for 2½ minutes or until cheese has melted.

PER SERVING	Calories: 240	Fat: 7 g
	Saturated fat: under 1 g	Fiber: 2 g
	Cholesterol: 9 mg	Sodium: 477 mg
	Calcium: 106 mg	Iron: 3.3 mg

RESOURCE: Judith Eaton and Karen Lefkowitz

Sloppy Joes with Texturized Soy Protein

Serves 4

7/8 cup boiling water
1 cup dry texturized soy protein
1 cup chopped onion
1 large green bell pepper, coarsely chopped
3 tablespoons soybean or canola oil
2 cups low-salt tomato sauce
1–1½ tablespoons chili powder
1 tablespoon low-sodium soy sauce
2 tablespoons sugar
Salt and pepper to taste
4 hamburger rolls, split in halves

1. Pour boiling water over the texturized soy protein and set aside.

2. In a large pan, sauté the onion and green pepper in the oil until they are tender, about 5 minutes.

3. Add the texturized soy protein and the rest of the ingredients. Simmer for 20 minutes.

4. Serve over split hamburger rolls.

PER SERVING	Calories: 371	Fat: 13 g
	Saturated fat: 2 g	Fiber: 8 g
	Cholesterol: 0	Sodium: 457 mg
	Calcium: 169 mg	Iron: 5 mg

RESOURCE: Adapted from a recipe developed by the United Soybean Board

Fusilli and Tofu with Sauce Verde

Serves 4

1 package (8 ounces) fusilli (corkscrew) pasta

1 package (10½ ounces) extra-firm low-fat tofu, drained and cut in ½-inch cubes

1–2 garlic cloves

½ cup chopped fresh parsley

½ cup chopped fresh cilantro

3 scallions

¼ cup grated Parmesan cheese, preferably fat-free cheese alternative

1 tablespoon olive oil

2 teaspoons sesame tahini

1 cup chopped raw broccoli

1. Prepare the pasta according to directions on the package. Drain and place in a medium bowl. Add the tofu.

2. Place the garlic, parsley, cilantro, scallions, cheese, olive oil and tahini in a food processor. Process until smooth. Add to the pasta and tofu.

3. Process the broccoli with an on/off motion until it is coarsely chopped. Add to pasta mixture. Toss well. Serve warm or cold.

PER SERVING	Calories: 329	Fat: 8 g
	Saturated fat: less than 1 g	Fiber: 1 g
	Cholesterol: 0	Sodium: 150 mg
	Calcium: 64 mg	Iron: 9 mg

RESOURCE: Judith Eaton and Karen Lefkowitz

Tofu Meatballs

Serves 4

1 large onion

1 cup chopped fresh curly parsley

2 packages (10½ ounces each) extra-firm low-fat tofu, drained

½ cup seasoned bread crumbs

½ cup egg substitute

½ teaspoon dried basil

½ teaspoon dried minced garlic

½ teaspoon dried oregano

½ teaspoon black pepper

½ teaspoon dry mustard

¼ teaspoon fennel seeds

¼ teaspoon ground nutmeg

¼ cup grated Parmesan cheese, preferably fat-free cheese alternative

1½ cups plus 3 tablespoons tomato sauce, preferably low-salt

¼ cup whole wheat flour

1. Preheat the oven to 350° F.

2. Place the onion and parsley in a food processor. Process until smooth.

3. Add the tofu, bread crumbs, egg substitute, herbs, pepper, mustard, fennel, nutmeg, cheese, and 3 tablespoons of tomato sauce. Process with on/off motion until ingredients are combined.

4. Form 16 balls the size of a walnut, then dust each with flour.

5. Coat nonstick baking pan with nonstick cooking spray. Place the balls in the pan and bake for 35 minutes.

6. Transfer balls to a large nonstick skillet that has been sprayed with nonstick cooking spray. Add the remaining tomato sauce, cover, and simmer 10 to 15 minutes or until sauce is hot.

PER SERVING	Calories: 237	Fat: 4 g
	Saturated fat: under 1 g	Fiber: 3 g
	Cholesterol: 0	Sodium: 436 mg
	Calcium: 140 mg	Iron: 5 mg

RESOURCE: Judith Eaton and Karen Lefkowitz

Tofu Cutlets Parmesan

Serves 6

1 onion, chopped
2 cups tomato sauce, preferably low-salt
1 teaspoon garlic powder
1 teaspoon dried oregano
2 packages (10½ ounces each) extra-firm low-fat tofu
½ cup egg substitute
¾ cup Italian-seasoned bread crumbs
4 ounces reduced-fat mozzarella cheese, grated
4 ounces Parmesan cheese, preferably fat-free cheese alternative, grated

1. Preheat the oven to 350° F.

2. Coat a large skillet with nonstick cooking spray, then sauté onion until wilted, about 3 minutes.

3. Put tomato sauce in a saucepan and add the onion and seasonings. Simmer for 15 minutes.

4. Meanwhile, slice each cake of tofu lengthwise into 3 pieces. Drain on paper towels for 15 minutes.

5. Heat a medium skillet. Dip each tofu slice in egg substitute, then coat with bread crumbs. Fry until delicately brown, about 3 to 4 minutes.

6. Line a baking pan with a little sauce and then layer in the cutlets, adding more sauce and some grated cheese between the layers, leaving some cheese for sprinkling on top. Bake for 20 minutes or until heated through and the cheese has melted.

PER SERVING	Calories: 188	Fat: 4 g
	Saturated fat: under 1 g	Fiber: 1.5 g
	Cholesterol: 7 mg	Sodium: 652 mg
	Calcium: 60 mg	Iron: 9 mg

RESOURCE: Judith Eaton and Karen Lefkowitz

Tofu Stuffed Pepper

Serves 5

1 cup cooked brown rice

5 green bell peppers

1 package (10½ ounces) extra-firm low-fat tofu, drained and diced

¼ cup low-sodium soy sauce

1 teaspoon garlic powder

2 small onions

1 celery stalk

2 tablespoons sesame tahini

1 jar (2 ounces) pimiento, drained and chopped
1 cup warm water
1 low-sodium bouillon cube

1. Cook the rice according to package directions.
2. Preheat the oven to 350° F.
3. Remove the seeds and membranes from the peppers, then cut each in half lengthwise.
4. Parboil the peppers for 10 minutes or until nearly tender.
5. While peppers are cooking, marinate the tofu in the soy sauce and garlic powder for 10 minutes.
6. Chop the onions and celery, then spray a skillet with non-stick cooking spray and sauté until tender, about 5 minutes.
7. Mix the rice, celery, and onion with the tahini and pimiento. Stuff the pepper halves with this mixture and then place peppers in roasting pan.
8. Dissolve the bouillon cube in the warm water and pour in roasting pan around the peppers. Bake for 10 to 15 minutes, or until peppers are soft and stuffing is hot.

PER SERVING	Calories: 328	Fat: 4 g
	Saturated fat: under 1 g	Fiber: 8 g
	Cholesterol: under 1 g	Sodium: 362 mg
	Calcium: 91 mg	Iron: 75 mg

RESOURCE: Judith Eaton and Karen Lefkowitz

Quinoa with Tofu

Serves 5

1 package (10½ ounces) extra-firm low-fat tofu

½ cup low-sodium teriyaki sauce

1 cup quinoa

2 cups water

2 teaspoons canola oil

1 teaspoon minced fresh ginger

1 onion, minced

3 celery stalks, chopped

2 tablespoons low-sodium soy sauce

1 cup frozen mixed vegetables, thawed

1. Cut the tofu into small cubes and marinate in teriyaki sauce for at least 30 minutes.

2. Rinse the quinoa several times by running fresh water over it in a pot and pouring through a strainer.

3. In a saucepan, bring 2 cups of water to a boil. Add the quinoa, reduce the heat, cover, and simmer until all water is absorbed, 15 to 20 minutes. Set aside.

4. Heat the oil in a large nonstick skillet. Add the ginger and stir. Add the onion and celery, and cook until lightly browned, about 5 minutes.

5. Add the cooked quinoa, soy sauce, and marinated tofu to the skillet. Stir once, cover, and cook for 5 minutes.

6. Add the vegetables. Cook for 2 minutes, covered, or until vegetables are heated through. Do not overcook.

PER SERVING	Calories: 215	Fat: 5 g
	Saturated fat: under 1 g	Fiber: 3 g
	Cholesterol: 0	Sodium: 470 mg
	Calcium: 53 mg	Iron: 8 mg

RESOURCE: Judith Eaton and Karen Lefkowitz

Crustless Onion-Mushroom Quiche

Serves 4

1 teaspoon canola oil

2 cups minced onions

2 cups minced fresh mushrooms, plus sliced mushrooms for garnish

¼ teaspoon salt

1½ cups egg substitute

½ cup skim milk or low-fat soy milk

1 package (10½ ounces) firm low-fat tofu

3 ounces grated reduced-fat Jarlsberg or Swiss cheese

1. Preheat the oven to 350° F.

2. In a large nonstick frying pan, heat the oil and cook the onions until lightly browned, about 5 minutes.

3. Add the minced mushrooms and cook over high heat for about 3 minutes. Sprinkle with salt and cook until the mushroom mixture is almost dry. Remove from pan and set aside.

4. In a food processor, blend the egg substitute, milk, and tofu. Add the cheese and mushroom mixture and stir well.

5. Spray a 10-inch quiche dish or pie pan with nonstick spray. Pour the mixture into the prepared pan and decorate the top

with mushroom slices. Bake for 40 minutes or until set. Let rest for 5 minutes before slicing.

PER SERVING	Calories: 191	Fat: 5 g
	Saturated fat: under 1 g	Fiber: 2 g
	Cholesterol: 12 g	Sodium: 428 g
	Calcium: 102 mg	Iron: 3 mg

RESOURCE: Judith Eaton and Karen Lefkowitz

Athenian Tofu

Serves 4

8 ounces orzo or other small pasta
2 cans (1 pound each) whole plum tomatoes, preferably low-salt
2 garlic cloves, chopped
1 teaspoon dried parsley, or 1 tablespoon fresh
1 teaspoon dried basil, or 1 tablespoon fresh
1 teaspoon dried oregano
1 package (10½ ounces) extra-firm low-fat tofu, crumbled
4 ounces feta cheese, crumbled
2 teaspoons capers, rinsed (optional)

1. Cook the orzo according to package directions. Keep hot.

2. Empty the canned tomatoes into a saucepan and bring to a boil, using a large spoon to cut tomatoes into smaller pieces.

3. Add the garlic, parsley, basil, oregano, and tofu. Reduce the heat and simmer for 10 minutes.

4. Add the feta cheese and capers. Simmer for 5 minutes and serve over hot orzo.

PER SERVING (EXCLUDING CAPERS)	Calories: 365	Fat: 8 g
	Saturated fat: 4.5 g	Fiber: 1.5 g
	Cholesterol: 25 g	Sodium: 414 mg
	Calcium: 230 mg	Iron: 4.5 mg

RESOURCE: Judith Eaton and Karen Lefkowitz

Okara Patties with Spicy Peanut Sauce

Serves 8

½ cup diced onion
1 garlic clove, crushed
¼ cup natural-style peanut butter
1 tablespoon honey
2 tablespoons lemon juice
½ teaspoon diced fresh ginger
Dash of cayenne pepper
1 tablespoon vinegar
1 cup water
1 tablespoon low-sodium soy sauce
2 packages (4 patties each) Natural Touch okara patty
4 cups shredded green cabbage
1 cup shredded carrot

1. Coat a large skillet with nonstick cooking spray, then sauté the onion until tender, about 5 minutes.

2. Add the garlic, peanut butter, honey, lemon juice, ginger, cayenne, vinegar, water, and soy sauce. Heat until boiling, and then reduce to a simmer.

3. Heat the okara patties according to package instructions.

4. Steam the cabbage and carrot in separate pans until tender.

5. Serve patties on a bed of the steamed vegetables, and pour sauce over top.

PER SERVING		
	Calories: 235	Fat: 14 g
	Saturated fat: less than 1 g	Fiber: 2 g
	Cholesterol: 24 mg	Sodium: 460 mg
	Calcium: 31 mg	Iron: less than 1 mg

RESOURCE: Worthington Foods, Inc.

Okara Pattie Foo Yong

Serves 4

1 package (4 patties) Natural Touch okara patty
1 teaspoon cornstarch
1 teaspoon sugar
1 teaspoon vinegar
1 tablespoon low-sodium soy sauce
½ cup water

1. Prepare the patties according to package directions.

2. Combine the ingredients for the sauce in a small saucepan. Cook over medium heat, stirring constantly, until the mixture thickens and boils.

3. Serve over the patties.

PER SERVING Calories: 169 Fat: 10 g
Saturated fat: less than 1 g Fiber: less than 1 g
Cholesterol: 0 Sodium: 521 mg
Calcium: 1.4 mg Iron: less than 1 mg

RESOURCE: Worthington Foods, Inc.

Tempeh Pizza

Serves 2

8 ounces tempeh
1 small onion, chopped
½ red bell pepper, chopped
½ cup sliced fresh mushrooms
½ teaspoon dry Italian seasoning
½ teaspoon dried basil
Salt and pepper to taste
½ cup meatless spaghetti sauce
2 ounces reduced-fat mozzarella cheese

1. Preheat the oven to 450° F.

2. Steam the tempeh for 15 minutes.

3. Coat a large skillet with nonstick cooking spray, and saute the onion and red pepper until onion is translucent, about 3 minutes.

4. Add the mushrooms and seasoning to the skillet, and continue cooking until the mushrooms are tender, stirring frequently, about 3 minutes.

5. Cut tempeh in half and place on baking sheet. Cover each piece with ¼ cup sauce, then half the vegetable mixture. Top each pizza with cheese.

6. Bake for 5 minutes or until the cheese is melted, or microwave on high until cheese is melted.

PER SERVING	Calories: 335	Fat: 15 g
	Saturated fat: 1 g	Fiber: 5.5 g
	Cholesterol: 20 g	Sodium: 475 mg
	Calcium: 122 mg	Iron: 3 mg

RESOURCE: Judith Eaton and Karen Lefkowitz

Busy Day Chili

Serves 6

2 cups texturized vegetable protein (TVP) with enough hot water to cover (about 1¾ cups)
1 onion, coarsely chopped
1 (15½ ounce) can kidney beans, rinsed and drained
1 cup canned corn
¼ cup chopped fresh parsley
3–4 tablespoons chili powder
3 teaspoons garlic powder
⅓ cup catsup
1 teaspoon low-sodium soy sauce
⅔ cup salsa or picante sauce
2½ cups water
½ cup shredded reduced-fat taco cheese

1. Cover the TVP with hot water and soak until moistened.

2. Coat a large, deep skillet with nonstick cooking spray and sauté the onion until lightly browned, about 5 minutes.

3. Add the TVP and the remainder of ingredients to the skillet. Adjust the seasonings to taste, and simmer the chili for at least 15 minutes to blend the flavors.

PER SERVING	Calories: 270	Fat: 4.5 g
	Saturated fat: under 1 g	Fiber: 14 g
	Cholesterol: 11 mg	Sodium: 994 mg
	Calcium: 153 mg	Iron: 5.5 mg

RESOURCE: Judith Eaton and Karen Lefkowitz

Sweet-and-Sour Hawaiian Tempeh

Serves 4

1 package (8 ounces) Lightlife Soy or Three Grain tempeh
1 teaspoon sesame or canola oil
2 carrots, sliced thin
1 cup unsweetened pineapple juice
3 tablespoons low-sodium soy sauce
2 garlic cloves, minced
2 teaspoons grated fresh ginger
1 tablespoon rice wine vinegar
1 tablespoon honey
1 medium red bell pepper, julienned
1 medium green bell pepper, julienned
1 cup broccoli florets, cooked
1 can (8 ounces) unsweetened pineapple chunks
2 teaspoons cornstarch dissolved in ¼ cup water
¼ cup slivered almonds

1. Steam the tempeh for 15 minutes.

2. Cut tempeh into eight 1½-inch squares. Cut each square in half to form 16 triangles, then slice each triangle crosswise so it is ¼-inch thick.

3. Heat the oil in a nonstick skillet and sauté the tempeh pieces for about 5 minutes on each side.

4. Add the carrots, pineapple juice, soy sauce, garlic, and ginger to the skillet. Simmer, covered, over low heat for 10 to 15 minutes.

5. Add the vinegar, honey, peppers, broccoli, and pineapple. Simmer, covered, for 5 minutes.

6. Add the cornstarch mixture and cook 1 minute longer.

7. Serve over steamed rice or noodles. Garnish with almonds.

PER SERVING	Calories: 292	Fat: 6 g
	Saturated fat: under 1 g	Fiber: 5 g
	Cholesterol: 0	Sodium: 840 mg
	Calcium: 78 mg	Iron: 2 mg

RESOURCE: Judith Eaton and Karen Lefkowitz

Quick-and-Easy Spinach Lasagna

Serves 5

1 cup texturized vegetable protein (TVP) and hot water to cover (about ⅞ cup)

3 cups prepared fat-free, meatless, low-salt spaghetti sauce or 3 cups homemade sauce

1 container (15 ounces) fat-free ricotta cheese

1 package (10 ounces) frozen chopped spinach, defrosted and squeezed dry.

¼ cup plus 2 tablespoons grated fat-free Parmesan cheese alternative

½ teaspoon dried oregano

2 egg whites

6 no-boil lasagna noodles, or regular lasagna noodles precooked and drained

1¼ cups shredded fat-free mozzarella cheese alternative or reduced-fat soy cheese

1. Preheat the oven to 350° F.

2. Cover the TVP with hot water and soak until moistened, then mix TVP with spaghetti sauce.

3. Mix the ricotta cheese, spinach, ¼ cup Parmesan cheese, oregano, and egg whites.

4. Spread a layer of sauce (about 1 cup) on the bottom of an 8-inch square pan. Place 2 noodles on the sauce, making sure that they do not touch the edges of the pan. Cover the noodles with more sauce, half the spinach mixture, and half the mozzarella. Repeat a layer of noodles, sauce, spinach, and cheese. End with a layer of noodles and sauce. Top with 2 tablespoons of Parmesan cheese.

5. Cover dish with foil and bake for 30 minutes. Uncover and bake for 10 more minutes. Let stand 5 minutes before serving.

PER SERVING	Calories: 314	Fat: 2 g
	Saturated fat: under 1 g	Fiber: 4.5 g
	Cholesterol: 20 mg	Sodium: 838 mg
	Calcium: 640 mg	Iron: 5 mg

RESOURCE: Judith Eaton and Karen Lefkowitz

Tempeh Reuben Sandwiches

Serves 4

8 ounces tempeh
¼ cup low-sodium soy sauce
8 slices rye bread
4 teaspoons prepared mustard
1½ cups sauerkraut, drained
4 ounces (4 slices) reduced-fat Swiss cheese

1. Slice the tempeh into quarters and cut each horizontally to make thin slices.

2. In a nonstick skillet, heat 2 tablespoons of the soy sauce and cook the tempeh on one side until brown, about 2 minutes. Add the remaining soy sauce, turn the tempeh, and cook over medium heat until lightly browned, another 2 minutes.

3. Toast the rye bread.

4. Spread mustard on each slice. Top bread with tempeh slice, sauerkraut, and Swiss cheese. Heat on high in microwave until the cheese has melted, about 1½ minutes.

PER SERVING	Calories: 362	Fat: 12 g
	Saturated fat: under 1 g	Fiber: 4 g
	Cholesterol: 15 mg	Sodium: 1825 mg
	Calcium: 132 mg	Iron: 4.5 mg

RESOURCE: Judith Eaton and Karen Lefkowitz

Barbecued Tofu

Serves 4

1 pound firm tofu, frozen and then defrosted
2 large onions, thinly sliced
1 cup barbecue sauce, preferably low-fat, low-sodium

1. Squeeze any excess water from the tofu. Slice the block of tofu across its short end into ¼-inch slices.

2. Place the onions in a baking dish and pour ¼ cup of barbecue sauce over them. Add the tofu and the remaining barbecue sauce. Let the tofu and sauce marinate in the refrigerator for several hours.

3. Preheat the oven to 375° F. Bake the tofu and onions for 20 to 30 minutes until the sauce is bubbling hot. (The tofu can also be cooked on the grill, brushing frequently with barbecue sauce.)

4. Serve over rice or stuffed into pieces of crusty French bread.

PER SERVING	Calories: 195	Fat: 6.4 g
	Saturated fat: 2 g	Fiber: 1.7 g
	Cholesterol: 0	Sodium: 240 mg
	Calcium: 35 mg	Iron: 1.6 mg

RESOURCE: Developed by the Soyfoods Association of America with funding from the United Soybean Board

Tofu with Condiments

This makes a great lunch or cold supper!

Serves 2

1 package (10½ ounces) firm or extra firm low-fat tofu
3 scallions
¼ cup chopped fresh cilantro
¼ red bell pepper
1 teaspoon roasted sesame seeds
¼ cup low-sodium soy sauce

1. Drain the tofu. Cut in half on the diagonal to form 2 triangles, then cut a pocket in each triangle.

2. Chop the scallion, cilantro, and pepper finely. Combine with sesame seeds.

3. Stuff half the scallion mixture in each piece of tofu.

4. Pour soy sauce over tofu pockets and marinate in refrigerator for 10 minutes before serving.

PER SERVING	Calories: 83	Fat: 2 g
	Saturated fat: under 1 g	Fiber: under 1 g
	Cholesterol: 0	Sodium: 743 mg
	Calcium: 52 mg	Iron: 11 mg

RESOURCE: Judith Eaton and Karen Lefkowitz

Sesame Tofu

Serves 2

¼ cup low-sodium soy sauce
2 tablespoons water
1 tablespoon vinegar
½ teaspoon sugar
½ teaspoon roasted sesame oil
1 scallion, chopped
½ teaspoon finely chopped fresh ginger
1 package (10½ ounces) extra-firm low-fat tofu
1 tablespoon sesame seeds

1. Mix the soy sauce, water, vinegar, sugar, sesame oil, scallion, and ginger in a bowl.

2. Cut the tofu in half horizontally and slice again into 4 pieces.

3. Pour the marinade over the tofu and refrigerate for at least 1 hour.

4. Preheat the oven to 450° F. Spray a baking sheet with nonstick cooking spray.

5. In a dry frying pan, roast the sesame seeds until lightly browned, a few seconds. Press seeds into the tofu and bake for 8 to 10 minutes or until lightly browned.

PER SERVING	Calories: 90	Fat: 4 g
	Saturated fat: under 1 g	Fiber: under 1 g
	Cholesterol: 0	Sodium: 455 mg
	Calcium: 39 mg	Iron: 11 mg

RESOURCE: Judith Eaton and Karen Lefkowitz

Noodle Pudding

Serves 9

1 package (10½ ounces) soft low-fat tofu, mashed
½ cup sugar
1 cup raisins
½ cup low-fat cottage cheese
½ cup nonfat sour cream
¼ cup skim milk or low-fat soy milk
1 teaspoon vanilla extract
1 cup canned, crushed unsweetened pineapple in juice, drained
½ cup egg substitute or 4 egg whites
1¼ teaspoons ground cinnamon
3 cups cooked cholesterol-free noodles or regular egg noodles (about 6 ounces dry)
¾ cups cornflake crumbs
2 tablespoons brown sugar

1. Preheat the oven to 350°F.

2. In a large bowl, combine the tofu, sugar, raisins, cottage cheese, sour cream, milk, vanilla, pineapple, egg substitute or egg whites, and ½ teaspoon cinnamon; stir well. Gently mix in noodles.

3. Spray an 8- or 9-inch square pan with nonstick cooking spray. Pour mixture into pan.

4. In a small bowl, mix cornflake crumbs, brown sugar, and ¾ teaspoon cinnamon. Spread evenly over the noodle mixture.

5. Bake for 1 hour or until set. Let stand 10 minutes before serving.

PER SERVING		
	Calories: 266	Fat: 1.6 g
	Saturated fat: under 1 g	Fiber: 1 g
	Cholesterol: under 1 g	Sodium: 196 mg
	Calcium: 63 mg	Iron: 4 mg

RESOURCE: Judith Eaton and Karen Lefkowitz

Tempeh-Lemon Broil

Serves 4

1 pound tempeh
1 large onion, sliced
Juice of 3 lemons
¼ cup olive oil
3 tablespoons low-sodium soy sauce
2 garlic cloves, minced

1. Cut the tempeh into 16 chunks. Place in a bowl with the sliced onion.

2. Mix the lemon juice, olive oil, soy sauce, and garlic. Pour mixture over tempeh and onion. Marinate for at least 3 hours in the refrigerator.

3. Preheat the oven to 400° F. Bake for 30 minutes in a roasting pan, basting with the marinade occasionally.

PER SERVING		
	Calories: 223	Fat: 15 g
	Saturated fat: 1 g	Fiber: 3 g
	Cholesterol: 0	Sodium: 307 mg
	Calcium: 63 mg	Iron: 2 mg

RESOURCE: Developed by the Soyfoods Association of America with funding by the United Soybean Board

Barbecued Grilled Tempeh with Onions

Serves 2

8 ounces tempeh

2 medium onions, thinly sliced

1 cup barbecue sauce, preferably low-fat, low-sodium

1. Preheat the oven to 350° F.
2. Cut the tempeh into 20 cubes.
3. Place the tempeh, onion slices, and barbecue sauce in a casserole sprayed with nonstick cooking spray. Cover and bake for 30 minutes. (The tempeh and onions can also be marinated in the barbecue sauce and then cooked on a grill.)

PER SERVING	Calories: 330	Fat: 9 g
	Saturated fat: 0	Fiber: 5 g
	Cholesterol: 0	Sodium: 1170 mg
	Calcium: 95 mg	Iron: 2 mg

RESOURCE: Developed by the Soyfoods Association of America with funding from the United Soybean Board

Tex-Mex Tempeh

A spicy filling for tacos, burritos, or tortillas.

Serves 4

1 package (8 ounces) Lightlife Corn-Jalapeño or Soy tempeh (see Note)

2 tablespoons canola oil
1 medium Spanish onion, in ½-inch cubes
2 garlic cloves, minced
1 teaspoon seeded and minced fresh chili pepper
1 teaspoon sea salt
1½ teaspoons ground cumin
1 tablespoon dried oregano
¼ teaspoon ground nutmeg
2 tablespoons tamari
1 tablespoon brown rice syrup
4 tablespoons tomato paste mixed with 1½–2 cups water

1. Grate or crumble the tempeh. Heat in a skillet and brown the tempeh for 2 minutes. Set aside.

2. In the same skillet, sauté the onion, garlic, chili pepper, and sea salt until onion is translucent, about 3 minutes.

3. Add the tempeh, cumin, oregano, nutmeg, tamari, sweetener, and tomato paste dissolved in water. Stir, cover, and gently simmer until liquid has evaporated, around 10 minutes.

4. Serve with burritos, tortillas, or taco shells.* Garnish with shredded lettuce, sliced tomatoes, avocado, olives, and cilantro.

Note: If using soy tempeh, use 3 garlic cloves, 1 whole fresh chili pepper, 2 teaspoons cumin, and ¼ cup each diced sweet red pepper and corn kernels.

PER SERVING	Calories: 206	Fat: 12 g
	Saturated fat: less than 1 g	Fiber: 3 g
	Cholesterol: 0	Sodium: 1174 mg
	Calcium: 87 mg	Iron: 3 mg

RESOURCE: Lynne Paterson, Lightlife Tempeh
* not included in analysis.

Rice and Tofu Loaf

Serves 4

½ pound firm tofu
1½ cups cooked brown rice
1½ tablespoons sesame oil
1 small onion, finely chopped
2 garlic cloves, minced
1 leek, cut in half lengthwise and diced
2 carrots, grated
¼ teaspoon Herbamare seasoning
2 teaspoons dried herbs (thyme, basil, etc.)
1 tablespoon low-sodium soy sauce
Handful of minced fresh parsley

1. Preheat the oven to 375° F.

2. Mash the tofu in a bowl.

3. Heat the oil in a skillet and sauté the onion, garlic, and leek until soft, about 3 minutes. Add Herbamare and dried herbs. Then stir in the carrots and continue to sauté for a few minutes until the vegetables soften.

4. Add the vegetables and remaining ingredients to tofu and mix well.

5. Transfer mixture to an 8½ x 4½-inch loaf pan or casserole dish that has been coated with nonstick cooking spray. Cover with foil and bake for 30 minutes.

6. Remove foil from loaf and bake for another 15 minutes, until the top becomes golden brown and slightly crisp. Allow to cool for about 20 minutes before removing from the pan and slicing.

PER SERVING (ANALYZED WITHOUT HERBAMARE)	Calories: 200	Fat: 8 g
	Saturated fat: 1 g	Fiber: 1 g
	Cholesterol: 0	Sodium: 270 mg
	Calcium: 109 mg	Iron: 5 mg

RESOURCE: Ana McIntyre

Tofu and Mushrooms

This makes a wonderful side dish as well as a main course.

Serves 4

1 can (14 ounces) clear beef broth, preferably low-fat, low-salt

½ cup dry red wine

3 tablespoons low-sodium Kikkoman soy sauce

2 tablespoons sugar

½ pound bite-size fresh mushrooms

1 package (14 or 16 ounces) firm tofu, cut in 1-inch cubes and drained

1½ tablespoons cornstarch

3 scallions, including tops, cut in 2-inch lengths

1. Set aside 2 tablespoons broth. In a large skillet, combine the remaining broth with wine, soy sauce, and sugar. Place in a saucepan and bring to a boil.

2. Add the mushrooms, reduce heat, and cover. Cook for 5 minutes.

3. Add the tofu, cover, and cook for 3 minutes.

4. Dissolve the cornstarch in the reserved broth, then add cornstarch mixture and scallions to the tofu mixture.

5. Cook, stirring gently, until thickened and translucent.

PER SERVING	Calories: 250	Fat: 10 g
	Saturated fat: 2 g	Fiber: 2 g
	Cholesterol: 0	Sodium: 830 mg
	Calcium: 248 mg	Iron: 13 mg

RESOURCE: Azumaya Inc.

Tofu Rice Stir-Fry

Serves 2

1 package (10½ ounces) extra-firm low-fat tofu, drained and cut into ½-inch cubes

¼ cup low-sodium soy sauce

¼ cup rice wine vinegar

1 tablespoon sesame oil

1 cup shredded carrots

1 cup sliced celery

½ cup sliced scallions

¼ cup sliced fresh ginger

1 cup cooked white rice

1. Combine the tofu, soy sauce, vinegar, and sesame oil. Marinate in refrigerator for a minimum of 1 hour.

2. Heat all the marinated ingredients in a wok. Add the carrots, celery and ginger. Stir-fry until vegetables are tender but still crisp, about 5 minutes.

3. Add the rice and stir-fry to heat through. Serve hot.

PER SERVING Calories: 337 Fat: 11 g
Saturated fat: 1 g Fiber: 5 g
Cholesterol: 0 Sodium: 1250 mg
Calcium: 140 mg Iron: 4 mg

RESOURCE: Mori-nu

Tofu Bouillabaisse

Serves 6

1 pound (16 ounces) firm tofu, drained
1 onion, chopped
1 large garlic clove, minced
2 tablespoons vegetable oil
½ pound white fish fillets (cod, scrod), cubed
1 can (4½ ounces) shrimp, rinsed and drained
1 can (12 ounces) or 1½ bottles (8 ounces each) clam juice
1 can (10¾ ounces) condensed chicken broth
½ cup dry white wine
1 large or 2 small tomatoes, chopped
⅓ cup chopped scallions
¾ teaspoon dried thyme
¼ teaspoon crumbled dried rosemary
1 bay leaf
Salt and pepper to taste (optional)

1. Cut the tofu into small cubes.

2. Sauté the onion and garlic in the oil in large saucepan until soft, about 3 minutes.

3. Add the fish and cook for 5 minutes.

4. Stir in the tofu and remaining ingredients, bring to boil, then simmer for 10 minutes to blend flavors.

PER SERVING		
	Calories: 264	Fat: 12 g
	Saturated fat: 2 g	Fiber: 54 mg
	Cholesterol: 54 mg	Sodium: 663 mg
	Calcium: 178 mg	Iron: 9 mg

RESOURCE: Azumaya Inc.

Chicken Tetrazzini

Serves 6

2⅓ cups canned low-salt chicken broth
2 packages (10½ ounces each) soft low-fat tofu
¼ cup neufchatel cheese
3 cups sliced fresh mushrooms
½ cup minced onion
1 tablespoon all-purpose flour
¼ cup grated Parmesan cheese, preferably fat-free cheese alternative
¼ cup dry sherry
¼ teaspoon salt
1½ teaspoons garlic powder
½ teaspoon black pepper
1½ cups frozen peas
1 jar (2 ounces) pimiento, drained and diced
½ pound spaghetti
2 cups chopped cooked chicken breast (about ½ pound)
1 teaspoon Worcestershire sauce

1. Preheat the oven to 350° F.

2. In food processor, mix the chicken broth, tofu, and Neufchatel cheese until smooth. Set aside.

3. Spray a large skillet with nonstick cooking spray. Sauté the mushrooms and onion over medium heat for 6 minutes.

4. Stir the flour into the mushroom mixture. Gradually add the tofu mixture. Bring to a boil and cook 5 minutes, stirring constantly.

5. Remove skillet from heat and stir in 2 tablespoons Parmesan cheese, sherry, salt, garlic powder, and pepper. Stir, add the peas and pimiento, then set aside.

6. Break the spaghetti into 4 lengths and cook according to package directions. Drain.

7. Stir spaghetti and chicken into the tofu mixture. Mix in the Worcestershire sauce, then pour into a 3-quart casserole coated with nonstick cooking spray. Sprinkle top with remaining Parmesan cheese.

8. Cover the casserole and bake for 20 minutes, then uncover and bake an additional 10 minutes. Let stand 5 minutes before serving.

PER SERVING	Calories: 302	Fat: 7 g
	Saturated fat: 2 g	Fiber: 3 g
	Cholesterol: 32 mg	Sodium: 233 mg
	Calcium: 97 mg	Iron: 25 mg

RESOURCE: Judith Eaton and Karen Lefkowitz

Chicken and Tofu Stir-Fry

Serves 6

1 pound extra-firm tofu, drained and cut in 3/4-inch cubes

1/4 cup low-sodium soy sauce

1 tablespoon cornstarch

1 whole chicken breast, skinned, boned, and cut into thin strips

1 tablespoon canola oil

1/2 pound broccoli, chopped

1 onion, cut into wedges

1 cup bean sprouts

2 garlic cloves, halved

6 cups cooked brown rice

1. Marinate the tofu in 2 tablespoons of the soy sauce for 10 minutes. Drain well.

2. Combine the used soy sauce with the cornstarch and marinate the chicken for 15 minutes.

3. In a large skillet or wok, stir-fry the tofu for 2 minutes in the oil until light brown (if using a wok, heat before adding oil).

4. Remove tofu and stir-fry the broccoli for 3 minutes. Add the onion and stir-fry 2 more minutes. Add the bean sprouts and stir-fry 1 minute.

5. Remove all the vegetables from the skillet or wok. Add more oil if necessary and toss in the garlic, stir-frying for 1 minute. Discard garlic and add chicken and marinade. Cook 2 to 3 minutes. Add remaining 2 tablespoons soy sauce, vegetables, and tofu; heat thoroughly.

6. Serve with cooked brown rice.

PER SERVING	Calories: 367	Fat: 7 g
	Saturated fat: 1 g	Fiber: 5 g
	Cholesterol: 24 mg	Sodium: 483 mg
	Calcium: 80 mg	Iron: 3 mg

RESOURCE: Adapted from a recipe developed by Bountiful Bean Soyfoods

Chicken Paprika

Serves 4

½ pound noodles, preferably no-yolks pasta
1 teaspoon canola oil
1 cup chopped onion
2 tablespoons Hungarian paprika
1½ cups fat-free, low-salt chicken broth
½ cup dry sherry
1 pound boneless and skinless chicken breast, cut into cubes
1 package (10½ ounces) firm low-fat tofu
1 tablespoon all-purpose flour

1. Cook the noodles according to package directions.

2. In a large, nonstick skillet, heat the oil, add the onions, and cook until lightly browned.

3. Add the paprika and cook for another minute. Add the chicken broth and sherry, then bring to a boil over high heat. Add the chicken cubes and cook over medium heat for 30 minutes.

4. Puree the tofu with the flour in a blender or food processor. Add to the skillet and bring to a boil. Serve over noodles.

PER SERVING Calories: 495 Fat: 12.5 g
Saturated fat: 2.5 g Fiber: under 1 g
Cholesterol: 94 mg Sodium: 264 mg
Calcium: 56 mg Iron: 4.5 mg

RESOURCE: Judith Eaton and Karen Lefkowitz

Beefy Tofu Enchiladas

Serves 8

1 package (10½ ounces) firm tofu, mashed
½ cup chopped onion
1 pound extra-lean ground beef, browned and drained
1 can (4 ounces) chopped green chilies
1 garlic clove, minced
1 teaspoon dried cilantro
½ teaspoon cumin seed
2 cups drained and diced tomatoes
8 8-inch flour tortillas
2 cups thick tomato salsa
1 cup shredded cheddar cheese, preferably reduced-fat, low-salt

1. Preheat the oven to 350° F. Lightly spray a 9 x 13-inch baking dish with nonstick cooking spray.

2. In a bowl, combine all the ingredients except the tortillas, salsa, and cheese.

3. Place ½ cup of the mixture in the center of each tortilla and roll up. Place in the baking dish, seam side down.

4. Pour the salsa over the enchiladas. Sprinkle with shredded cheese. Cover pan with aluminum foil and bake for 25 to 30 minutes.

PER SERVING	Calories: 370	Fat: 17 g
	Saturated fat: 4.5 g	Fiber: 1 g
	Cholesterol: 50 mg	Sodium: 600 mg
	Calcium: 290 mg	Iron: 4 mg

RESOURCE: Soy Ohio

Meat Loaf

Serves 4

½ pound extra-lean ground beef
½ pound extra-firm low-fat tofu, mashed
½ cup bread crumbs, preferably from whole wheat bread
½ package dry onion soup mix
2 egg whites
1 carrot, grated
1 can (8 ounces) tomato sauce, preferably low-salt

1. Preheat the oven to 350° F.

2. In a bowl, mix the beef, tofu, bread crumbs, soup mix, egg whites, and carrot with ½ can tomato sauce.

3. On a broiler pan (or use a loaf pan [8½ x 4½-inch]), shape the mixture into a loaf. Top with remaining tomato sauce and bake for 1 hour or until cooked through.

PER SERVING	Calories: 265	Fat: 10 g
	Saturated fat: 4 g	Fiber: 1 g
	Cholesterol: 60 mg	Sodium: 261 mg
	Calcium: 60 mg	Iron: 9 mg

RESOURCE: Judith Eaton and Karen Lefkowitz

Breads and Breakfasts

Peach Breakfast Soufflé

Serves 4

1 package (8.4 ounces) Creamy Original Vitasoy soy milk
1 large egg and 1 egg white
1 teaspoon orange juice concentrate
1 teaspoon honey or maple syrup
½ teaspoon each grated lemon and orange zest
¼ teaspoon ground cinnamon
2 large slices whole-grain bread
2 fresh peaches, 1 chopped and 1 sliced

1. Preheat the oven to 375° F. Coat a small 2-quart casserole with nonstick cooking spray.

2. Beat together all the ingredients except the bread and sliced peach.

3. Lay one slice of bread in the casserole and pour half the liquid over it. Top with half the sliced peaches, then the other slice of bread. Cover with the remaining liquid and finally with the remaining sliced peaches.

4. Bake for 60 minutes or until the top is golden and firm to the touch. Let cool before serving.

PER SERVING	Calories: 107	Fat: 3g
	Saturated fat: less than 1g	Fiber: 1g
	Cholesterol: 53 mg	Sodium: 93 mg
	Calcium: 43 mg	Iron: 1 mg

RESOURCE: Vitasoy, Inc.

Toffins

Makes 12 muffins

1 cup old-fashioned rolled oats
¾ cup whole wheat pastry flour
¼ cup soy flour, preferably defatted
2 teaspoons baking powder
½ teaspoon salt
1 teaspoon ground cinnamon
¼ teaspoon ground cloves
½ cup chopped walnuts
½ cup raisins
1 large apple, chopped
¼ cup banana, mashed
¼ cup maple syrup
1 package (10½ ounces) soft low-fat tofu

1. Preheat oven to 350° F. Spray a muffin tin with nonstick cooking spray.

2. Combine the oats, flours, baking powder, salt, cinnamon, cloves, walnuts, raisins, and apple.

3. Process the banana, maple syrup, and tofu in a food processor until completely blended.

4. Combine the tofu mixture with the dry ingredients until moistened. Pour into muffin cups and bake for 35 to 45 minutes, or until a toothpick inserted in center comes out clean. Cool completely before eating.

PER SERVING:	Calories: 158	Fat: 5 g
	Saturated fat: under 1 g	Fiber: 2 g
	Cholesterol: 0	Sodium: 153 mg
	Calcium: 83 mg	Iron: 1 mg

RESOURCE: Judith Eaton and Karen Lefkowitz

Zucchini Bread

Makes 2 loaves of bread (about 13 slices each)

1 cup all-purpose flour
1¼ cups whole wheat flour
¾ cup soy flour, preferably defatted
2 teaspoons ground cinnamon
1 teaspoon baking powder
1 teaspoon baking soda
1 cup raisins
½ cup egg substitute or 4 egg whites
⅓ cup unsweetened applesauce
1 package (10½ ounces) soft low-fat tofu, pureed
1 cup packed brown sugar
2 teaspoons vanilla extract
2 cups finely shredded zucchini

1. Preheat the oven to 350° F. Coat two 8 x 4-inch loaf pans with nonstick spray.

2. Combine the flours, cinnamon, baking powder, baking soda, and raisins in a bowl.

3. In a large bowl, beat the egg substitute or egg whites until foamy. Combine eggs with applesauce, tofu, brown sugar, and vanilla. Stir in zucchini.

4. Add the flour mixture and mix until well blended.

5. Pour batter into prepared pans and bake for 55 minutes or until a toothpick inserted in center comes out clean.

6. Cool pans on a rack for 10 minutes. Remove loaves from pans and cool thoroughly before slicing.

PER SERVING (1 SLICE)		
	Calories: 113	Fat: 1 g
	Saturated fat: under 1 g	Fiber: 1 g
	Cholesterol: 0	Sodium: 61 mg
	Calcium: 27 mg	Iron: 1 mg

RESOURCE: Judith Eaton and Karen Lefkowitz

Eastern Omelet

This simple omelet can easily be dressed up with the addition of sliced mushrooms, peas, chopped spinach, or bean sprouts.

Serves 4

1 cup drained diced Azumaya Kinugosihi soft tofu
10 egg whites, beaten
⅓ cup low-fat milk
3 tablespoons chopped scallion
½ teaspoon salt
⅛ teaspoon pepper
1 tablespoon butter or margarine or nonstick cooking spray
Soy sauce or light tamari to taste (optional)

1. Combine the tofu, egg whites, milk, scallion, salt, and pepper in a bowl.

2. Melt the butter or shortening in a large skillet or coat with nonstick cooking spray.

3. Add the egg-tofu mixture and cook slowly. Run a spatula around the edge, lifting to allow any uncooked portion to flow underneath. When the eggs are set, fold in half and turn out onto a warmed serving platter. Serve with soy sauce if desired.

PER SERVING	Calories: 112	Fat: 5 g
	Saturated fat: 1 g	Fiber: 1 g
	Cholesterol: 0	Sodium: 419 mg
	Calcium: 55 mg	Iron: 1 mg

RESOURCE: Adapted from a recipe developed by Azumaya Inc.

Apple Pancakes

Serves 4; makes 12 pancakes

3 tablespoons sugar
½ teaspoon ground cinnamon
¼ teaspoon ground nutmeg
⅛ teaspoon salt
1 cup all-purpose flour
1 tablespoon soy flour
2 teaspoons baking powder
¾ cup soy milk
1 teaspoon vanilla extract
2 tablespoons margarine, melted and cooled
1 tart apple, peeled, cored, and grated

1. Mix the sugar with the cinnamon, nutmeg, and salt. Blend sugar mixture with the flours and baking soda.

2. In a separate bowl, whisk together the soy milk, vanilla, and margarine. Pour over the dry mixture and blend well. Fold in the apples.

3. Pour ¼ cup of batter onto a hot nonstick griddle or pan. Cook for about 2 minutes on one side, or until bubbles appear on surface, then flip and cook for another minute or until heated through.

4. Serve topped with applesauce and maple syrup.

PER SERVING (PER PANCAKE)	Calories: 80	Fat: 2 g
	Saturated fat: less than 1 g	Fiber: less than 1 g
	Cholesterol: 0	Sodium: 85 mg
	Calcium: 60 mg	Iron: less than 1 mg

RESOURCE: Developed by the Soyfoods Association of America with funding from the United Soybean Board

Banana Pancakes

Serves 4

1 cup all-purpose flour
½ cup soy flour, preferably defatted
1 teaspoon salt
1¾ teaspoons baking powder
3 tablespoons soybean oil
1¼ cups plain soy milk
2 bananas, thinly sliced
Fresh, sliced fruit or maple syrup (optional)

1. Sift together the flours, salt, and baking powder.

2. In a separate bowl, mix the oil and milk. Add quickly to the dry ingredients, stirring just to blend. Add the bananas and stir into the batter with just a few strokes.

3. Pour batter by ¼ cupfuls onto a lightly oiled griddle and cook for 2 to 3 minutes or until bubbles begin to form on the pancakes. Then flip and cook on the other side for 1 to 2 minutes. Serve with fresh fruit or maple syrup.

PER SERVING	Calories: 363	Fat: 12 g
	Saturated fat: 2g	Fiber: 5 g
	Cholesterol: 0	Sodium: 553 mg
	Calcium: 62 mg	Iron: 3 mg

RESOURCE: United Soybean Board

Desserts

Chocolate Tofu Berry Whip

An unbelievably delicious dessert.

Serves 3

1 package (10½ ounces) firm or extra-firm low-fat tofu

1 cup raspberries or any other berries, frozen and unsweetened

½ cup fruit-sweetened blackberry jam (14 calories per teaspoon)

1 teaspoon vanilla extract

1 teaspoon fresh lemon juice

1 tablespoon cocoa powder

1. Place the tofu, berries, jam, vanilla, lemon juice,and cocoa powder in a food processor. Process until smooth.

2. Spoon into parfait glasses and serve.

PER SERVING	Calories: 182	Fat: 1 g
	Saturated fat: less than 1 g	Fiber: 2 g
	Cholesterol: 0	Sodium: 95 mg
	Calcium: 30 mg	Iron: 8 mg

RESOURCE: Judith Eaton and Karen Lefkowitz

Chocolate Chip Cookies

Makes approximately 80 cookies

1¾ cups all-purpose flour
¾ cup soy flour, preferably defatted
½ cup Dutch-process cocoa
1 teaspoon baking soda
1 jar (2½ ounces) strained prunes (baby food)
2 teaspoons vanilla extract
2 tablespoons light corn syrup
1 cup granulated sugar
1 cup packed light brown sugar
½ cup soft low-fat tofu
¼ cup skim milk or low-fat soy milk
½ cup miniature chocolate chips

1. Preheat the oven to 350° F. Spray cookie sheets with non-stick cooking spray.

2. In a large bowl, mix the flours, cocoa, and baking soda and set aside.

3. In another bowl, mix the prunes, vanilla, corn syrup, sugars, tofu, and milk. Beat with an electric mixer at high speed until well blended. Add this mixture to the dry mixture and blend well. Add chocolate chips and mix.

4. Drop a teaspoonful of batter at a time onto the cookie sheet, leaving about 1 inch between the cookies. Bake for 10 minutes. Let cool on rack.

PER COOKIE	Calories: 45	Fat: under 1 g
	Saturated fat: under 1 g	Fiber: under 1 g
	Cholesterol: under 1 g	Sodium: 18 mg
	Calcium: 7 mg	Iron: under 1 mg

RESOURCE: Judith Eaton and Karen Lefkowitz

Chocolate Cream Pie

Serves 8

PIE CRUST

¼ cup low-fat margarine
1¼ cups graham cracker crumbs

FILLING

1 cup sugar
1 envelope unflavored gelatin
⅓ cup Dutch-process cocoa
¾ cup skim milk or fat-reduced soy milk
1 package (10½ ounces) firm light tofu, pureed
1 teaspoon vanilla extract

1. Melt the margarine, then add to bread crumbs and blend well.

2. Press crumbs into a 9-inch pie pan. Chill at least 15 minutes.

3. In a medium saucepan, mix the sugar, gelatin, and cocoa. Slowly stir in the milk and let stand 5 minutes.

4. Cook over medium heat, stirring constantly, until the mixture comes to a boil and gelatin is dissolved. Add the tofu and vanilla; stir until well combined.

5. Pour into prepared crust and chill several hours until firm.

PER SERVING	Calories: 255	Fat: 6 g
	Saturated fat: under 1 g	Fiber: under 1 g
	Cholesterol: under 1 g	Sodium: 200 mg
	Calcium: 50 mg	Iron: 2 mg

RESOURCE: Judith Eaton and Karen Lefkowitz

Tofu Brownies

Gooey and delicious.

Makes 16 brownies

¾ cup all-purpose flour
½ cup soy flour, preferably defatted
⅓ cup Dutch-process cocoa
1¼ cups sugar
¼ teaspoon baking soda
2 tablespoons cornstarch
1 jar (2½ ounces) strained prunes (baby food)
½ cup soft low-fat tofu, pureed
2 teaspoons vanilla extract
2 tablespoons light corn syrup
¼ cup miniature chocolate chips or chopped walnuts (optional)

1. Preheat the oven to 350° F. Coat an 8-inch square pan with nonstick cooking spray.

2. Sift together in a large bowl the flours, cocoa, ½ cup sugar, baking soda, and cornstarch. Mix well.

3. In another bowl, with an electric beater or whisk, mix the prunes, tofu, vanilla, corn syrup, and ¾ cup sugar until well blended.

4. Combine wet ingredients and dry ingredients; mix until smooth. The batter will be very thick. Fold in optional chips or walnuts.

5. Bake for 25 minutes. Cool and cut into 16 squares.

PER SERVING		
	Calories: 120	Fat: under 1 g
	Saturated fat: under 1 g	Fiber: under 1 g
	Cholesterol: 0	Sodium: 24 mg
	Calcium: 10 mg	Iron: 1 mg

RESOURCE: Judith Eaton and Karen Lefkowitz

Tofu Strawberry Cheese Cake

Serves 8

CRUST

1 cup graham cracker crumbs

2 tablespoons canola oil

1 tablespoon brown sugar

FILLING

¾ cup egg substitute

1 package (10½ ounces) extra-firm low-fat tofu, drained and cut into small pieces

¼ cup maple syrup

2 tablespoons lemon juice

1 teaspoon vanilla extract

3 ounces fat-free ricotta cheese

TOPPING

2 cups fresh strawberries

½ cup all-fruit strawberry preserves

1. Preheat the oven to 325° F.

2. Mix the graham cracker crumbs with the oil and brown sugar. Press into a 9-inch pie pan.

3. In a food processor, whip the egg substitute. Add the tofu, syrup, lemon juice, and vanilla. Blend until smooth. Add the ricotta cheese and blend until smooth.

4. Pour filling into pie crust and bake for 45 to 55 minutes. Cool for 5 minutes.

5. Cover pie with fruit. Heat the preserves, then pour over strawberries. Chill for several hours before serving.

PER SERVING	Calories: 205	Fat: 5 g
	Saturated fat: under 1 g	Fiber: under 1 g
	Cholesterol: 3 mg	Sodium: 160 mg
	Calcium: 65 mg	Iron: 4 mg

RESOURCE: Judith Eaton and Karen Lefkowitz

Creamy Spritzer

Serves 2

½ cup vanilla-flavored soy milk, preferably low-fat

½ cup orange juice

1 cup sparkling water

1. Blend the soy milk and orange juice in a blender.

2. Pour mixture over ice and add sparkling water.

PER SERVING	Calories: 60	Fat: 12 g
	Saturated fat: 2 g	Fiber: 0
	Cholesterol: 0	Sodium: 54 mg
	Calcium: 60 mg	Iron: 3 mg

RESOURCE: United Soybean Board

Tofu Pumpkin Pie

Serves 8

1 can (16 ounces) pureed pumpkin
¾ cups sugar
½ teaspoon salt
1 teaspoon ground cinnamon
½ teaspoon ground ginger
¼ teaspoon ground cloves
1 package (10½ ounces) soft tofu processed in a blender until smooth
1 9-inch unbaked pie shell

1. Preheat the oven to 425° F.

2. Cream the pumpkin and sugar. Add the salt, spices, and tofu, mixing thoroughly.

3. Pour mixture into pie shell and bake for 15 minutes. Lower the heat to 350° F. and bake for an additional 40 minutes.

4. Chill before serving.

PER SERVING	Calories: 195	Fat: 6 g
	Saturated fat: 2 g	Fiber: 2 g
	Cholesterol: 0	Sodium: 240 mg
	Calcium: 35 mg	Iron: 2 mg

RESOURCE: Developed by the Soyfoods Association of America with funding from the United Soybean Board

Strawberry Fluff

Serves 4

1 package (10½ ounces) soft tofu, drained

3 tablespoons honey

2½ cups frozen strawberries, thawed and drained

1. In blender or food processor, combine the tofu and honey. Blend until smooth and creamy.
2. Add the strawberries, ½ cup at a time. Allow some berries to remain in chunks.
3. Pour into stemmed glasses. Chill and serve.

PER SERVING	Calories: 125	Fat: 2 g
	Saturated fat: less than 1 g	Fiber: 2 g
	Cholesterol: 0	Sodium: 25 mg
	Calcium: 35 mg	Iron: 1.5 mg

RESOURCE: Missouri Soybean Board

Super-Moist Carrot Cake

Serves 16

2 cups plus 2 tablespoons whole wheat flour

2½ teaspoons ground cinnamon

1½ teaspoons ground nutmeg

1½ teaspoons baking soda

¾ teaspoon ground cloves

1 package (10½ ounces) soft tofu, drained

½ cup vegetable oil

⅔ cup honey

2 teaspoons vanilla extract

2¼ cups finely shredded carrots

1 can (8 ounces) unsweetened crushed pineapple in juice, drained

1. Preheat the oven to 350° F.

2. In a medium bowl, combine the flour, cinnamon, nutmeg, baking soda, and cloves. Set aside.

3. In a food processor or blender, combine the tofu, oil, honey, and vanilla. Blend until smooth.

4. Pour the tofu mixture into the flour mixture. Mix until dry ingredients are moist, then add the carrots and pineapple. Stir until well blended.

5. Pour mixture into an ungreased 8-inch square baking pan. Bake for 40 to 45 minutes or until a toothpick inserted in the center of the cake comes out clean. Serve slightly warm.

PER SERVING	Calories: 180	Fat: 8 g
	Saturated fat: 1 g	Fiber: 2.5 g
	Cholesterol: 0	Sodium: 125 mg
	Calcium: 24 mg	Iron: 1.1 mg

RESOURCE: Missouri Soybean Board

Vanilla Pudding

Serves 3

½ cup sugar
2 tablespoons cornstarch
⅛ teaspoon salt
1½ cups plain soy milk
1 teaspoon vanilla extract

1. In a saucepan, stir together the sugar, cornstarch, and salt. Slowly add the soy milk, stirring to prevent lumps.

2. Bring the mixture to boil. Lower heat to a simmer, stirring constantly for about 5 minutes, until mixture is thick and creamy. Remove from heat.

3. Stir in the vanilla and pour into dessert cups. Chill until mixture sets.

PER SERVING	Calories: 145	Fat: 2 g
	Saturated fat: less than 1 g	Fiber 1 g
	Cholesterol: 0	Sodium: 78 mg
	Calcium: 4 mg	Iron: Less than 1 mg

RESOURCE: Developed by the Soyfoods Association of America and the United Soybean Advisory Board

"Piña Colada"

Serves 4

1 package (10½ ounces) soft tofu
1½ large ripe bananas
2 cups unsweetened pineapple juice
½ teaspoon coconut extract
2 tablespoons sugar or to taste

1. In a blender or a food processor, combine all the ingredients. Whip until smooth.

2. Cover and chill in the refrigerator for at least 1 hour before serving, or serve over crushed ice.

PER SERVING (ANALYZED WITHOUT COCONUT EXTRACT)	Calories: 178	Fat: 2.4 g
	Saturated fat: less than 1 g	Fiber: 1.6 g
	Cholesterol: 0	Sodium: 161 mg
	Calcium: 41 mg	Iron: 1 mg

RESOURCE: Mori-nu

Low-Cal Chocolate Mousse

Serves 10

¾ cup honey or fruit sweetener
½ cup cocoa powder
3 teaspoons vanilla
2 packages (10½ ounces each) low-fat firm tofu, drained

1. Heat honey or fruit sweetener for 90 seconds in a microwave. Pour over cocoa powder. Add vanilla. Stir until smooth.

2. Blend tofu until smooth. Add chocolate mixture and continue blending for 1 minute. Chill 1 to 2 hours.

PER SERVING	Calories: 114	Fat: 1 g
	Saturated fat: 0	Fiber 0
	Cholesterol: 0	Sodium: 53 mg
	Calcium: 19 mg	Iron: 1 mg

RESOURCE: Mori-nu